Long-Awaited Pregnancy

A Healthy Way of Getting Pregnant and Improving Fertility. The First Book of an Expectant Mother

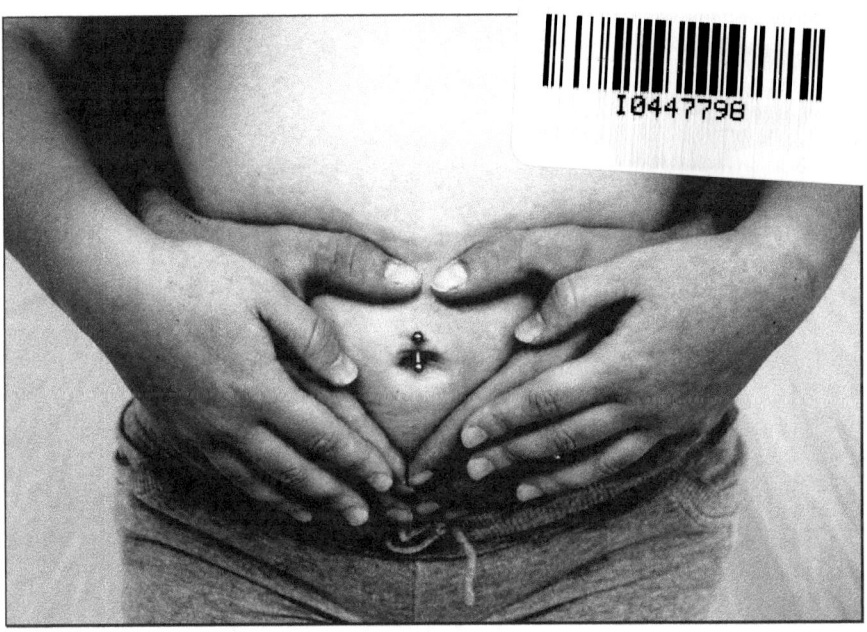

I0447798

Many women all over the world do want to experience motherhood; however, not everyone is blessed with the opportunity due to the lack of knowledge on how to successfully conceive one. This obstacle can now be overcome through the lessons and anecdotes presented by the book. Through this book, you will learn what proper steps to take months before conceiving a baby.

Contents

Part 1: Are You Ready to Make a Baby?

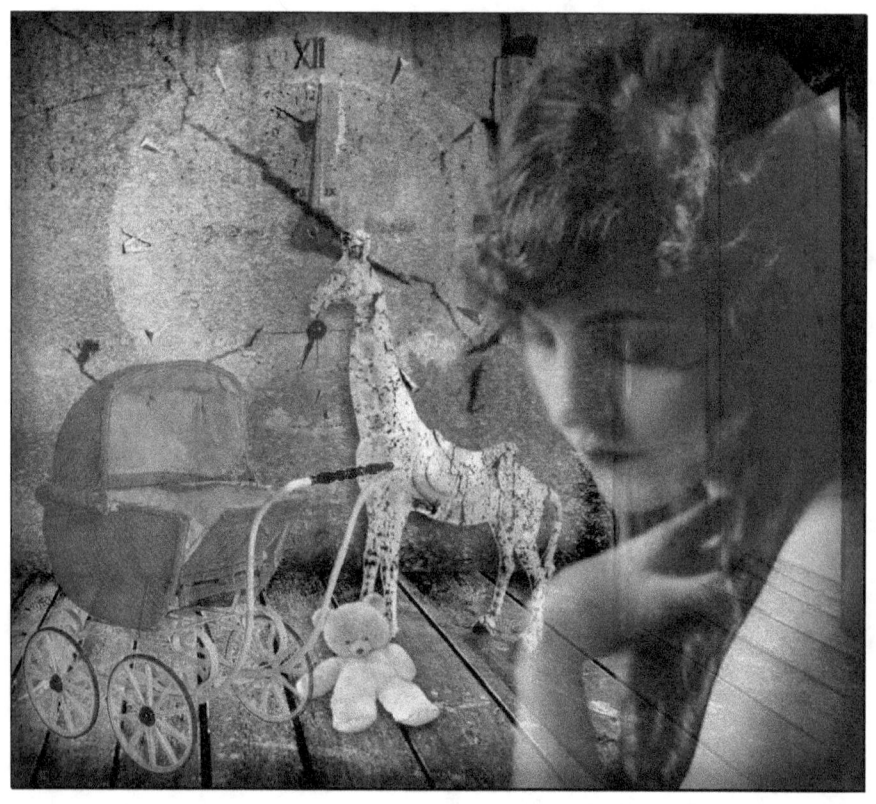

Chapter 1: Prepping For a Long-Awaited Pregnancy

Pregnancy is a great task for any woman to go through. It is a great physical, mental, and emotional process that every woman should prepare for. That is why a planned pregnancy is ideal because then the woman together with her partner and the rest of her family are all ready to welcome a soon-to-be-born new addition to the family. Now, if women acknowledge that pregnancy is not a walk in the park, how does one prepare for it?

Prepping before expecting is not something you can work overnight. It takes time for any woman to prepare to conceive – and this does not only mean preparing the body. Preparation for pregnancy is three-fold: first, the woman needs to make sure that her body is physically ready to conceive. Second, the woman needs to make sure that she is emotionally ready to conceive. And last, the woman needs to make sure that she is financially ready to conceive. In addition to the woman's preparation, preparation should also be undertaken by her husband because it is her husband's physical, emotional, and also financial support that will make this entire process easier.

To make the preparation a bit more doable, here are 15 things to do before even considering pregnancy:

1) *Go to an OB-GYNE*

If you want to have a successful pregnancy and safe delivery, you need to pay your OB-GYNE a visit. If you still do not have one, ask your close friends or relatives who to go to. It is important that you have an open and comfortable professional relationship with your doctor because your doctor will see you through this entire process.

If you already have been seeing one, then all the better. You need to tell your OB-GYNE that you are planning to get pregnant so he/she can give a timeline of when your body is ready to conceive. If you are taking birth control pills, your doctor will also have to advise you when to stop it and when to start trying to conceive.

Your husband should also consult with your doctor or with a urologist just to find out if his body is healthy enough and if his reproductive system is producing healthy sperms.
Having a clear understanding of your current physical, medical state will make your pregnancy plans safer and more doable.

2) *Start Sweating*

Follow a daily exercise regime at least six months before getting pregnant. There is no need for further explanation; exercise is healthy for the body, but it is, more importantly, necessary for women (and men) who want conceive. Studies suggest that women who exercised more regularly are more likely to conceive than women who live sedentary lives. This is most especially true for women who wish to undergo IVF treatment to conceive.

Exercise helps balance the body's release of hormones as well as regulates and optimizes the functions of all muscles and organs. Moreover, exercise syncs the performance of all the important organs directly related to conception. Through exercise the brain stimulates the production of healthy eggs and normalizes the release of sex hormones which makes the body more ready to conceive.

You do not need to do strenuous exercises just to keep you at an optimal state. Daily 30-minute walks or 15-minute jogs is good enough to ready your body for that much-anticipated pregnancy. If there is no time to exercise due to work, make sure you exert more effort in doing extra steps every day. For example, instead of taking the escalator or elevator, take the stairs just to elevate your pulse rate. Or increase your allotted time to clean the house or to tend the yard. Anything you can do to sweat and keep that heart healthy is good enough to prepare your body for pregnancy.

3) *Attain your Ideal Weight*

In conjunction to following a daily exercise regime, attaining your ideal weight is an important step in prepping for pregnancy. Staying within your ideal weight will mean that your BMI is also within normal levels. Keeping within normal BMI levels will lessen any pregnancy risks for you and your baby. Having a normal BMI will also increase your chances of getting pregnant.
If you are overweight, then you must cut down on the usual fatty, fast-food kind of diet that you are used to. If you are underweight, then you must increase your intake of healthy food.

4) *Consult a Nutritionist*

Weight loss or weight gain may just be easier to achieve when supported by experts in the field of nutrition. About six months before planning to conceive, it is best to pay a visit to a nutritionist. Your nutritionist will most likely check your glucose, sodium, and potassium levels as well as checks your current BMI level, weight, body mass, and body fat. All of this information will paint a picture of your current health and will give your nutritionist enough background to provide a well-thought meal plan.

5) *Get More Sleep*

While some women rack up on sleep only upon pregnancy, it is actually healthier to invest in more sleep months prior to getting pregnant. Sleep directly affects the amount of hormones released by the body. If a woman gets enough to sleep every night, about 7 to 8 hours, it increases her chances for healthier fertility periods. Studies even suggest that women who have regular sleeping patterns, sleeping at the same time and waking up at the same time, are 15% more likely to conceive than women who have erratic sleep patterns and get less than 7 hours of sleep every day. Conversely, women who get more than 10 hours of sleep or who sleep late in the evening and wake up late in the morning may have difficulty conceiving due to the irregular sleep pattern. The brevity or the length of a woman's sleep gives clues as to what lifestyle the woman is living. Those who spend less time in bed may mean that they have an active nightlife while those who spend excessive time in bed may mean having a sedentary lifestyle. The best solution to get the suggested 7 to 8 hours of sleep is to have enough daily exercise, eating a well-balanced diet, cutting down on night outs, and decreasing stress.

6) *Invest in Vitamins*

There is no harm in increasing your vitamin intake for as long as you also have the go signal of your family doctor. Studies suggest that increasing vitamin intake at least 3 months before trying to get pregnant will increase chances of conceiving. If you already adjusted your diet but still lack essential vitamins from what you are eating, then you may need to take the necessary supplements. Pregnant women need to increase intake of calcium and iron, so even before you get pregnant increase your consumption of food rich in iron and calcium like dark leafy vegetables and dairy products respectively. If your consumption isn't enough, then you can get iron and calcium tablets.

Another important supplement that will improve chances of getting pregnant and will ensure the healthy pregnancy is folic acid. Daily intake of about 400mcg of folic acid is enough to lessen pregnancy risks like defects in fetal developments. In addition, would be expecting moms need to increase intake of vitamin A, C, and, D.

Finally, even would be fathers need to increase intake of vitamin C, folic acid, and zinc to produce healthy sperm cells.

Do not forget to consult your family doctor prior to taking these supplements. It is still best to have yourself checked before increasing your vitamin and mineral intake.

7) *No Ifs and Butts*

If you want to conceive, to get through pregnancy with ease, and to give birth to a healthy baby, then you need to quit smoking. Smoking does not only affect your lungs; the tar, nicotine, and smoke that you inhale go to your bloodstream and are carried to the other organs in your body. Your reproductive organ is directly affected by this bad habit. A lot of studies prove that smoking causes infertility to many women. In addition, women who smoke up their chances of experiencing miscarriage, stillbirth, and preterm delivery. Even children who are born of smoking mothers have greater chances of having health problems like respiratory and heart issues.

If you do not smoke but your husband does, then you need to tell him to stop right away. Second-hand smoke is even worse than smoking itself. Aside from its negative effect on you, smoking can also increase your husband's chances of being infertile or worse impotent. So if you really want to have a healthy family, you really need to quit smoking – no ifs and butts!

8) *Say No to Alcohol*

If you are a heavy drinker, then you need to cut down your alcohol consumption. Although there is no clear study stating what level of alcohol consumption gives a negative effect on women who wish to get pregnant, saying no to alcohol is still the right thing to do. Your partner should do the same sacrifice as you too. Alcohol may have an indirect effect on your future child so to be on the safe side, do not drink too much first.

Occasional drinking may be acceptable while you are still trying to conceive but keep it down to a glass of wine.

9) *Limit your Night Outs*

One of the ways to keep yourself away from temptations like alcohol, cigarettes, fatty food, and other vices is to limit your night outs. If you are a party animal, then you know that it is quite difficult to say no to temptations. The only way to avoid all these is not to go out at all. Your friends will understand your situation for sure and will be totally supportive of your decision to take a rain check. Not only are you avoiding such vices, but you are also avoiding erratic sleep patterns by skipping night outs. You may have a fear of missing out but this sacrifice is all worth it once you find out that you are expecting.

10) *Say Yes to Shots*

No, this does not refer to tequila shots. The shots that you need to say yes to are the medical shots that you need to ensure safe and healthy pregnancy. For sure your family doctor or OB-GYNE will suggest what vaccinations you need to update to avoid any diseases that may affect your reproductive system or your baby. Some of the shots that you may need are flu vaccine, chicken pox vaccine, Tdap vaccine, and Measles, Mumps, and Rubella vaccines. It is highly recommended to take such vaccinations at least three months prior to conceiving because these vaccinations have live viruses that may affect the fetus.

11) *Say Cheese*

You need have to have that perfect set of teeth with a sparkling smile but it is important to see your dentist months before trying to get pregnant. Believe it or not, gum disease directly affects fetal health and development. More than 50% of women with gum disease end up giving birth to an underweight infant or giving birth earlier than expected. To avoid such unfortunate events, a visit to your family dentist is necessary. It is better to have yourself checked than regret after giving birth.

12) *Lower Caffeine Consumption*

You often hear pregnant women or breastfeeding mothers take a pass on caffeine-rich drinks because it has a negative effect on their babies; however, it is also true that soon-to-be expecting women also need to avoid such drinks at least a month before getting pregnant. Too much consumption of caffeine may lead to fertility issues, miscarriages, preterm delivery, and underweight infants. So before you take a swig of what is inside your glass or mug, make sure that what you are drinking does not contain caffeine. You need to avoid caffeinated drinks such as coffee, carbonated drinks, chocolate, tea, and energy drinks. Caffeine can also be present in some pain medication so double check before taking it.

13) *Take Advice from Experienced Mothers*

Apart from the physical preparation, women also need to prepare for this milestone mentally, emotionally, and spiritually. Most especially for first-time mothers, the preparation, is more important because expectations go as far as what are read in books and what are advised by doctors. To add a more personal touch, you can seek advice from experienced mothers who can guide you prior to your pregnancy until you give birth. It is best to talk to your own mother, mother-in-law, older sister, best friend, and even a colleague. Be open with them about your hesitations, fears, and anxieties as well as your excitement, eagerness, and enthusiasm about being pregnant and giving birth. Your relatives' and friends' advice and personal anecdotes about their own experiences will give you a clearer picture of what pregnancy and motherhood are all about. It will also give you a gauge of how prepared you are for this great responsibility.

14) *Check your Emotional State*

Stress may affect the body's ability to conceive because of the mix signals sent by the brain to other endocrine glands in the body. One of the glands that may directly be affected by stress is your ovary. Your ovaries may irregularly produce eggs which can affect your menstrual cycle. If you do not know the changes in your menstrual cycle, you will have a more difficult time figuring out whether you are fertile or not. Aside from affecting your fertility, stress may cause illnesses which can delay your chances of getting pregnant.

It is important to keep your stress levels to a minimum especially when preparing for pregnancy. Once you are pregnant, your body secretes a lot of hormones which may result in mood swings. So if you are stressed when you conceive, you might not be able to handle the rollercoaster emotional ride that pregnancy may cause and this can lead to post-partum depression.

The only way to counter this is always to be positive and avoid being in situations that may affect your happy disposition.

15) *Start Saving*

When you want to raise a family, you need to be practical. Preparing for pregnancy is not just about being healthy and feeling positive; it is also about being able to financially support your pregnancy, childbirth, and most especially child rearing. To be honest, all these processes cost a lot of money, and you need to be practical and thrifty enough to be able to save for your future. You should talk to your partner and plan a new budget scheme that will appropriate enough funds for expenses connected to your future pregnancy and childbirth. You may also want to explore getting medical insurance that will cover childbirth.

Chapter 2: Your Weight Before Pregnancy

As mentioned in the first chapter, staying in your ideal weight is important in optimizing your chances of conceiving. There really is a direct link between your weight and your fertility. If you are currently overweight, your reproductive system may have difficulty producing ova which will lessen the chances for ovulation. Moreover, being overweight may result in excess production of estrogen. This overproduction is triggered by the excess fat cells present in the body. For this reason, overweight and obesity are great hindrances to your pregnancy plans.

How do you know if you are overweight or obese?

One way to find out if you are overweight or obese is knowing your BMI or Body Mass Index. Body Mass Index is the ratio of your body fat in comparison to your height. BMI is what nutritionists, doctors, and gym instructors use as a basis for your diet plan or exercise plan. A BMI of over 25 means a person is an overweight while a BMI of over 30 means a person is obese. Keeping the BMI between the normal range of 18.5 to 24.9 increases the chances of normalizing ovulation; hence optimizing fertility.

You really do not need to visit a nutritionist just to know your BMI. You can calculate your own BMI at home just by using your bathroom weighing scale and your wall-mounted height ruler. If your weighing scale measures by pounds, simply divide your weight by 2.2 to convert it to kilograms. If your ruler height measures by inches, simply multiply your height by 0.025 to convert it to meters. Square your height in meters.

After getting this, divide your weight in kilograms to the square of your height in meters.

Now that you have a clear picture of your health through your BMI, you can now take necessary steps to help lower it until it reaches the normal level.

Does being underweight affect fertility as well?

Most people assume that only overweight women experience difficulty conceiving, however, this is also true for underweight women. Women who fall under the ideal weight range are reported to have problems in ovulating due to irregular menstrual cycle. Moreover, being underweight means that the body does not have enough fat that triggers the production of estrogen. This results in hormonal imbalance which results to infertility

What activities can you do to lose weight?

There are many ways to achieve your ideal weight, but the most effective way to lose weight is by doing physical activities. Exercise helps improve the body's metabolism which promotes burning off excess calories and fat. In addition, exercise promotes the production of hormones that boosts one's emotional state which can also help in conception.

Here are reminders that can help you lose that extra pound at the same time increase your chances of getting pregnant:

1.   Moderate your Exercise

Light and moderate exercises are highly recommended for women who want to get pregnant. Doing too many strenuous activities may have an adverse effect on your hormones and reproductive system so just remember that, although you want to lose that extra weight, you also want to conceive. The best exercise that you can do daily is brisk walking or jogging.

Spend at least 30 minutes every day walking or jogging around your community and you will see positive results in a month's time. Not only will you see your weight change, but you will also feel more active and more positive. This positivity will also affect your partner and may also encourage him to join you in your new daily routine.

2. Mix it Up

Doing the same exercise every day may lessen your chances of achieving your ideal weight because of boredom. Once in a while, you need to mix it up and change your exercise routine. Changing your exercise routine does not only keep you motivate but also improves your blood circulation which promotes healthy production of egg cells. You can maybe try aerobics every other week or try joining Zumba classes at least once a week. Just remember not to overdo it. Keep your exercise to 30 minutes to an hour every day.

3. Try Yoga

More than being a form of exercise, yoga promotes good breathing technique that can be a great preparation for childbirth. In addition, yoga helps reduce stress as it starts and ends with meditation. Finally, yoga burns that extra fat without having to do the strenuous physical task that may affect your reproductive system.

Chapter 3: A Healthy Eating

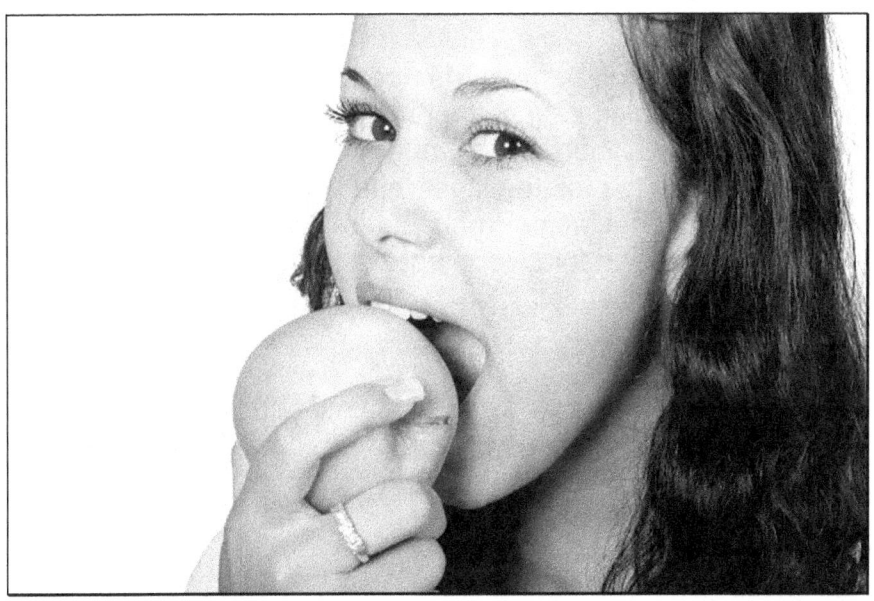

Following a healthy diet is important in preparing your body for pregnancy. Having a healthy diet plan should not only be applicable to underweight and overweight women, but also to women who are in perfect weight. The food that you need take prior to your pregnancy must be rich in iron, calcium, folate, and other vitamins and minerals to improve fertility and enhance pregnancy. This chapter will explain the different kinds of nutrients the body needs prior to pregnancy.

Folate

Folate is a type of vitamin B or B9 that women need when planning to conceive. The reason why folate is important for women is the fact that it prevents neural tube defects and brain defects during the development of the fetus in the womb. Folate can be found in the following food:

- *Muesli or Healthy Cereals*

Just a half cup of muesli is already packed with 100mcg of folate which is ¼ of the recommended daily folate allowance. When buying muesli or cereals, make sure you check the folate, sugar, and fiber content written in the nutritional facts. Purchase the brand that has the most fiber and folate content but has less sugar.

- *Broccoli*

Broccoli is not only rich in vitamin C, but it is also packed with folate. Just steam these green flowers, and half a cup of it will give you 50mcg of folate.

- *Spinach*

Do not be deceived by Popeye's favourite vegetable. It does not only give you energy, but it also is packed with fibers, beta-carotene, and folate. Just blanch these dark green leaves, and you will receive at least 40 mcg per serving.

- *Eggs*

This commonly misconstrued food is actually rich is vitamins, protein, and folate. When purchasing eggs at a nearby grocery, choose the organic ones or the ones rich in omega 3.

The suggested daily intake of folate is 400mcg. Although it might be difficult to take in the daily suggested intake through your meals, you can take the synthetic form of folate called folic acid. Consult with your OB-GYNE to make sure your folic acid intake is within the recommended levels.

Iron

Equally as important as folate, iron is important in normalizing a number of red blood cells and hemoglobin of women. Since women menstruate monthly, there is a greater chance that a lot of women are anemic. Unfortunately, anemia may cause infertility due to poor blood circulation. The solution to this problem is to increase intake of food rich in iron.

• *Liver*

It may have an odd metallic taste but liver is actually packed with iron. When taken in moderation, it may be enough to supply the body of the much-needed dosage. Be careful not to eat too much of it though because these dark meats are also rich in cholesterol which may also affect your ovulation.

• *Shellfish*

Shellfish are one of the best sources of iron. Try adding several oysters, clams, mussels, or scallops to your diet and you may not have to deal with anemia anymore. Aside from anemia, shellfish also prevent the formation of goiter, the swelling of the thyroid gland.

• *Beans*

Beans are more known to be packed with protein but unknown to a lot of people, beans are also rich in iron. Make it a point to add a little of chickpeas, tofu, soybeans, lentils, and white beans to your meals. These power seeds can also replace red meat to help you lose that extra weight.

Calcium

Calcium is essential in strengthening bones and prevention of muscle cramps. Women are preparing to get pregnant need calcium because it promotes the healthy development of embryos. Consuming the right amount of calcium may increase the chances of a healthier pregnancy because your body's calcium will form a protective layer around the developing embryo. Even your husband can benefit from taking calcium. Calcium, in men, helps produce healthy sperms that can swim swiftly through the alkaline-filled reproductive system of women.

- *Milk*

Milk is the best source of calcium. A glass of milk is packed with about 200mg of calcium or one-fifth of the daily recommended intake. It is best to consume milk at bed time because it also helps build and relax your muscles which will aid in better sleep.

- *Yogurt*

If you are trying to lose weight, you may want to prioritize taking yogurt over milk. A serving of plain yogurt is filled with more than 200mg of calcium. Aside from having less fat than milk, yogurt also contains probiotics that eliminate bad bacteria.

- *Salmon*

This pinkish fish is not only rich in omega 3 but also rich in calcium. The regular canned salmon in brine is packed with almost half the daily recommended dosage of calcium. Make a healthy salmon sandwich once in a while to boost your body's calcium content.

Part 2: A Pregnancy Process

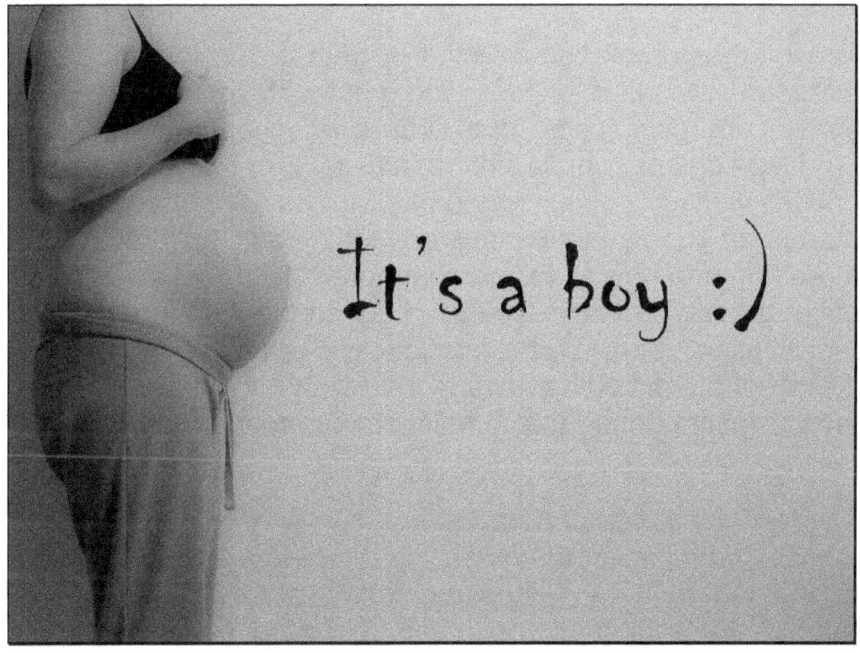

Chapter 4: The Biology Process of New Life

There are several processes that occur during the intercourse. Unknown to most, the biology of baby making is as complex as the pregnancy stage itself. It is not simply the intimate connection of a couple but the biological synergy and synthesis of two individual genetic structures to form a unique genetic strain. It is quite amazing and at the same time unbelievable to be able to see and understand the entire process behind the baby making. Knowing this scientific fact can open your eyes to the brilliance of the human body; hence be more appreciative of this blessing as well as be more mature of the responsibility called reproduction.

The Female Reproductive System

The internal female reproductive system is mainly composed of a uterus, a pair of ovaries, and a pair of fallopian tubes. The ovaries are microscopic, oval-shaped endocrine glands that produce eggs or ova. At birth, females internally have millions of eggs waiting to ripen and to be fertilized. By puberty, the number of eggs a female has dropped to less than half a million. In a female's lifetime, there are more or less 400 eggs out of the million that will be used during the female's reproductive years. These reproductive years commence at the onset of the first menstruation and end at the very last menstruation, during the completion of menopause.

The fallopian tubes or oviduct are a pair of microscopic tunnels that connect the ovaries to the uterus. Once an ovum or egg has matured, it goes out of the ovary and travels through the fallopian tube. The inner lining of each fallopian tube is filled with tiny hairs called cilia, which gently pushes and transports the ovum from the ovary to the uterus. When these tiny hairs do not function correctly, the egg may get stuck inside the tube and can potentially be fertilized by a male sex cell which will result to an ectopic pregnancy.

The uterus is a pear-shaped empty sac that holds the mature egg for several days. If the egg is fertilized, then the uterus will be the nurturing environment where the fetus will grow and develop. If the egg is not fertilized after the grace period, the uterus, together with some of its thin lining, will flush out the unfertilized egg and these will all come out in the form of blood during menstruation.

The ovaries, fallopian tubes, and the uterus all connect to the external parts of the female reproductive system. The lower part of the uterus connects to the cervix, a flexible tunnel that connects the internal reproductive system to the vagina. The normal width of a woman's cervix is about 2cm; however, during childbirth, it can expand to 10cm. Finally, the vagina is a muscular passageway that acts as the opening where sperm cells enter and as the canal where the infant can exit.

Understanding the Menstrual Cycle

You might be wondering why the understanding menstrual cycle is vital in the baby making process, the truth is knowing your menstrual cycle is the best basis for determining your fertile days and your infertile days. Women need to understand this to either prevent or permit pregnancy.

For women who experience menstrual cycles in an almost perfect rhythm and timing to a 28-da cycle, these are the normal phases that your bodies go through before, during, and after menstruation:

- *The Menstrual Phase*

  The menstrual phase starts on the first day of menstruation and ends about four days after. During this phase the uterus sheds a part of its inner lining together with the unfertilized egg and the blood vessels in and around it. Normal blood loss can measure up to 70ml per day. Anything more than that should be consulted with an OB-GYNE. During the first couple of days, it is normal for women to experience abdominal cramps and lower back pain due to the muscle contractions in the cervix area.

- *The Follicular Phase*

The follicular phase starts at the same time as the menstrual phase; however, the difference is this phase lasts until after 13 days after the first the day of menstruation. During this phase the brain sends signals to the ovaries to start producing another egg. As this happens, the female reproductive hormone called estrogen is released to control the production of follicles that can develop the eggs. Because of this hormone, the body is able to stop overproduction of eggs; thus only one follicle within one of the ovaries is allowed to mature and to develop an egg. When the strongest follicle is determined by the body, the uterus will form another lining that will soon welcome the fertilized egg.

While this phase is developing, it is believed that these 10 to 13 days are the least fertile days of a woman who has a 28-day menstrual cycle.

- *The Ovulation Phase*

The ovulation phase happens halfway through the 28-day cycle which is on the 14th day. During this day, the brain releases another signal to tell the dominant follicle to release the egg to the uterus. The brain also sends signals to the cervix to produce thick layers of nutrients to strengthen and protect potential sperms that can be fertilized the egg. This phase commences the fertile period of the woman.

- *The Luteal Phase*

The luteal phase starts a day after the ovulation phase. This phase is crucial because this is the phase when the egg stays in the fallopian tube and waits for sperm to fertilize it. If no sperm fertilizes it within 24 hours, the egg may lose its strength because it will move from the fallopian tube to the uterus. If the egg still doesn't get fertilized within the next few days, the uterus will shed the new lining and will commence the next menstrual phase.

The Male Reproductive System

It is equally important to know the male reproductive system when planning to get pregnant. Fertilization is the conception of the male and the female sex cells; therefore it is paramount to know your partner's anatomy and determine whether your fertile phase coincides with his.

Contrary to the female reproductive system, the majority of the organs that make the male reproductive system are found outside the body. The reason why these organs need to be located externally is due to its vulnerability to heat. Since the normal body temperature of about 36°C is too hot for sperms to survive, the male body evolved in such a way that its sperm-producing glands are just hanging outside the body. The external organs of the male reproductive organs are the testicles, scrotum, and penis.
The testicles are a pair of endocrine glands that produce the male sex hormone called testosterone. This hormone travels within the testicles and goes to seminiferous tubules. These tubes, triggered by testosterone, produce millions of sperm cells. Similar to the female ovaries, most men have a pair of testicles although men can still reproduce with only one functioning testicle.

The penis is a muscular organ that is used for both expelling urine and semen. Unlike the female anatomy, both urine and semen exit at the same passageway called the urethra. During sexual intercourse, the shaft of the penis receives more blood flow which stiffens the muscles surrounding the organ. This allows the penis to penetrate the female's vagina and also shuts down the urinary tract to just allow the ejaculation of semen. Semen is a protein-rich whitish fluid that contains millions of sperm cells. This fluid fortifies as well as lubricates the sperms to make traveling inside the acid-rich vagina and cervix more bearable. Once one out of the million sperms meets the female egg, the process of fertilization takes place.

The Biology of Sexual Intercourse

Now that you know your own anatomy as well as your partner's reproductive organs, it is vital to know what biologically transpires during sexual intercourse. A lot of people enjoy the arousal brought about by sexual intercourse but unknown to most people, this arousing sensation is what makes sexual intercourse not only enjoyable for the couple involved but also productive for the couple's biological makeup.

During sexual intercourse, the body goes through different phases that make the experience ecstatic yet fruitful. There is no definite duration for each of the phases because it varies per person. Furthermore, it is unlikely for both male and female to transition through each phase at the same time. Despite the difference in timing, the entire sexual act is made possible through the understanding of each other's body languages.

1.   Stimulation

The first phase of sexual intercourse is called stimulation. Couples enter the stimulation phase during foreplay. It is the time when the couple's brains release signals to other glands to secrete hormones like adrenaline, dopamine, and oxytocin. These hormones are what makes sexual intercourse enjoyable and arousing.

Aside from the release of such hormones, the male and female bodies undergo a few changes. First, the muscular systems of the couple stiffen due to the intense blood flow. To answer the need for faster blood flow, the heart pumps faster as breathing accelerates. Since blood surges through the different parts of the body, extremities start to stiffen – nipples become erect. The woman's clitoris and the man's penis swell and become erect as well. Finally, the woman's vagina begin to excrete a natural lubricant while the male's testicles balloons to produce sperm and fluid.

2. Plateau

The second phase is called plateau not because the sexual act stagnates but because the body maintains the changes that happened during the first phase. This means that high heart rate, accelerated breathing, erect penis and clitoris, and production of hormones are all maintained if not even intensified. During this phase, the female pleasure points become highly delicate and sensitive and may even be painful when stimulated. To counter the pain, the clitoris sinks behind the skin to avoid friction. Meanwhile, the man's testicles retreat further inside the scrotum as if pressing towards the penis. This is to increase pressure once the body reaches orgasm. As the body moves closer to the next phase, more muscles in the extremities stiffen – toes and fingers may contort uncontrollably.

3. Climax

The third phase is called climax. Although much awaited by both parties, this phase lasts for only a few seconds, unlike the other phases which may last for minutes, sometimes even an hour. During the climax, the male or the female reaches orgasm. Although it is quite impossible for any couple to reach climax at exactly the same time, both can still reach climax at any point during sexual intercourse. During the climax, the penis feels muscular contractions at its base to ejaculate semen. Meanwhile, for women, the vaginal muscles contract to naturally bring the semen towards the uterus. During this phase, the muscles involuntarily contract and breathing are at its peak.

4. <u>Resolution</u>

The last phase is called resolution. This is the phase when the body suddenly relaxes, and blood flow immediately goes back to normal. This results in the penis and clitoris going back to its normal size. The body feels fatigued but at the same time, with the rush of hormones, feels accomplished and happy. This is the phase when couples rest while cuddling. Women can easily go back to the stimulation phase a few seconds after reaching the resolution phase. In fact, women can reach climax immediately after this phase. However, men need more time to recuperate and may take more time in this phase than women. Older men may even take an hour or so to go back to stimulation phase.

Fertilization Process

What happens inside the body after sexual intercourse? If the male ejaculated inside the female's vagina, there is the chance that one of the male's sperms will meet the female's fertile egg. It is actually not as simple as it sounds. The travel from the vagina to the uterus and up to the fallopian tube is quite a difficult feat for those microscopic sperms.

The difficult journey of the male's sperms immediately begins right after the climax phase. So while you and your partner are still resting and cuddling in bed, inside your body a gun start for a sperm obstacle race has begun. The first hurdle that the sperms need to be overcome is the acid in the vagina. Some women have a more acidic vaginal fluid than others so just with this first hurdle, hundred thousands of sperm are expected to die. Sperms that are stronger survive and swim towards the cervix, the second hurdle. The cervical wall is covered in the viscous fluid which is hard to swim through especially for weak sperms. This fluid becomes thicker when the female is least fertile but it becomes more liquid when the female is fertile. Only the strongest sperms can swim through this cervical fluid and it is expected that a few hundred thousands of sperms will have perished at this point. After the getting through the cervical fluid, the surviving sperms have a world-like empty space to conquer. Once they enter the uterus, they need to locate the fallopian tube and attach to the egg. This is when a lot of sperms get lost, trapped, and die. Only about a dozen of sperms will luckily locate the egg. Once they locate the egg, the sperms need to attach itself to it and try to penetrate the protective layer before it can really fertilize the egg. The very first sperm that penetrates through the protective layer will come into contact with the egg and this commands the egg to put another protective layer to lock in the winning sperm and to not allow other sperms to get through. After 24 hours, the fertilization process begins. After three or so days, the fertilized egg will travel down to the uterus and will attach itself to the wall where it will get its nutrients for the next 36 weeks.

Chapter 5: The Ovulation and The Conceiving

Knowing when you are ovulating is the best method to increase your chances of getting pregnant. You must know and understand what happens in your body so that you can easily calendar your ovulation period. For those are not familiar with the different ways to predict ovulation, expect this chapter to open your eyes on the different signs that tell if you are ovulating.

Definition of Ovulation

Before going to the different ways to know your ovulation period, it is essential to understand what the word ovulation means. The word "ovulation" comes from the Latin word ovule which literally translates to the small egg. From its etymology, ovulation can be defined as the process that involves the release of a small egg from the ovary to the fallopian tube. Ovulation is one phase of the menstrual cycle that takes place about 14 days after the first day of menstruation for women with a 28-day cycle.

Methods to Determine Ovulation Period

Women who know how to track their ovulation period have greater chances of getting pregnant than women who do not have any knowledge of their ovulation period. There are several ways to figure out when you are ovulating:

- *Ovulation Calendar*

One of the best ways to keep track of your ovulation period is by following an ovulation calendar. If it is your first time to make your own ovulation calendar, start the process by predicting when the first day of your upcoming menstrual cycle will be. Unfortunately, this method is only effective for women who have regular 28-day menstrual cycles. If, for example, your next menstrual cycle will start on the 20th day of the month, count back 12 days. This will be the 8th day of the month. This day will be the last day of your ovulation period. From the 8th day, count back another five days. This means that the 3rd day of the month is the start of your ovulation period. Therefore, the 3rd to the 8th days of the month are your most fertile days.

For women who have 30-day menstrual cycles, you need to count back 15 days from the first day of your next menstruation. For women who have 25-day menstrual cycles, you need to count back ten days from the first day of your next menstruation. Women who have shorter menstrual cycles have short ovulation periods; however, it doesn't follow that women with longer menstrual cycles have longer ovulation periods.

There are actually many applications available online that can help women keep track of their ovulation period. Download one of these free applications so you can easily calendar the days you should consummate with your partner.

• *Body Temperature Chart*

Another way of determining your ovulation period is by taking down your basal body temperature first thing every morning. Basal body temperature can be measured by a special thermometer called the basal body thermometer. This thermometer can detect slight changes in the body's basal temperature. Women, during the first half of their menstrual cycle, have normally lower body temperature.

Their body temperature will reach its lowest at the onset of ovulation and then will immediately spike up after the ovary has released an egg. The reason for this sudden increase in temperature is due to the increase of the hormone called progesterone. Its side effect is the sudden increase of body temperature.

Unlike the calendar method which can immediately be utilized, the body temperature chart needs to be completed charted a couple of months ahead before a pattern can be drawn from it. Once you see a pattern when your temperature dips and then suddenly increases, this marks your ovulation period.

- *Fluid Discharge Chart*

In between your menstrual cycles, you will notice that there are days when you feel sudden discharges from your vagina. As weird as it sounds, taking note of the consistency of these discharges can help you determine your ovulation period. A couple of days after your last menstruation day, you will undergo a dry spell. This means that your cervix is not creating much mucus because it knows that it is not necessary because the body is not fertile at all. However as your cycle moves closer to ovulation phase, the cervix will start to produce mucus to cover its walls. Some of the excess mucus escape through the vagina. A few days before your ovulation period begins, you will notice that the discharges are somewhat dry, sticky but not as fluid. However, once you get nearer your ovulation period, the mucus will become clearer and comparable to the consistency of egg whites. If you put the discharge between your index finger and thumb and pull it apart, it should be able to form a string across your fingers. This kind of discharge marks the onset of ovulation. This method may be a little icky, but it is one method that actually works. To have a more accurate result, make a discharge chart parallel to a body temperature chart and draw your ovulation pattern from there.

- *Ovulation Predictor Stick*

If you do not mind spending money every time you pee, then you can purchase the ovulation predictor stick. Each stick costs around $20. Pee on the stick and if it shows a positive sign, it means you are two days away from ovulation and you have enough time to plan your intimate time with your partner. These sticks are proven effective; however, instead of peeing on one a few days after your menstruation and throwing away money every time, you can lessen the expense by still charting either your ovulation calendar, basal body temperature, or your discharge. Think of these sticks as the icing to your ovulation period charts – its main purpose is to confirm the validity of your charts. Once you have confirmed that you have predicted the correct pattern, you need not use the stick anymore.

Choose one or two from the methods explained above and you will have a better chance of getting pregnant. You can involve your partner in reminding you and encouraging you to continue your daily charting so that you can time your sexual intercourse and you can conceive in no time. For sure you partner is eager to get you to bed so you will not have any problems getting enough motivation from him.

Chapter 6: What You Need to Know About Fertility

Have you tried getting pregnant for more than a year and have not found success? You may need to have yourself checked to see if you have fertility issues. Do not worry about such issues because there are several common fertility issues that can be treated by the right doctor.

Ovulation Issue

Some women do not know that they have problems ovulating not until they want to get pregnant. Ovulation issues commonly stem from the irregular release of hormones that signal ovulation. This usually happens in women who have irregular menstrual cycles. When the release of hormones is all mixed up, the ovaries do not get the right signal when to produce and release an egg.

In order to solve ovulation issues, your OB-GYNE will most likely prescribe hormone pills that will try to normalize your menstrual cycle. Once your menstrual cycle is regular, then it could mean that your ovulation period has also been regularized. It may take some time to solve this issue, but your patience and diligence are needed to successfully solve the problem

Fallopian Tubes Issue

Some cases of infertility are attributed to fallopian tubes issue. Some women may have blocked fallopian tubes due to a bacteria called Chlamydia. When the fallopian tubes are blocked, this means that there is no way for the sperms to meet the egg. Likewise, there is no way for the egg to reach the uterus.

This fertility issue can be treated by your OB-GYNE. You may be prescribed oral medication to treat the infection that caused the blockage. Others may result in the laparoscopic procedure, but it all depends on the severity of the blockage.

Uterus Issue

Some cases of infertility are due to a thickened lining of the uterus. This issue is called endometriosis. When the uterus lining is thicker than normal, there is no way that a fertilized egg can successfully attach itself to the uterus. Sometimes it attaches itself to the wrong part of the reproductive system, which causes miscarriage or unsuccessful pregnancy. Women who are not aware of having endometriosis usually experience frequent menstruation or heavy menstruation.

In order to solve this issue, your OB-GYNE may recommend you to take oral medications to regulate your hormones. However, if the lining is really thick, you may go through a procedure that will take away excess lining from your uterus.

There is no harm in having a check up to determine if you do have fertility issues or not. Sometimes it is the fear of the unknown that prevents women from visiting their doctors, but early detection is key to be able to solve such issues while it has not progressed yet.

Chapter 7: Successfully Conceive a Baby

A lot of couples read and research on what sexual positions can optimize chances of conceiving. Some even go as far as timing male ejaculation with the hopes of conceiving a male or a female baby. To be honest, none of these have the scientific basis. There is no particular sexual position that can optimize conception nor is there a perfect timing to procreate a specific gender. The truth of the matter is females only have a few fertile days to conceive and within those fertile days, there is only less than 40% chances of successful fertilization. This rate is under the assumption that there are no reproductive system issues for both male and female adults. Do not feel discouraged by the rate of conception because there are pre-intercourse practices that you can do to help your body to successfully conceive a baby.

Prior to Having Sex

What should couples do before having sex to increase chances of procreating? This is probably one of the most asked questions by a lot of hoping couples. Of course, the first thing that any couple should do prior to having sex is to think of non-strenuous activities that will lower their stress levels. Stress levels can directly affect your reproductive system. When your mind is overwhelmed by stress, your body takes that negatively which may affect your menstrual cycle. You do not want that to happen because you will have a harder time estimating your fertile phase. Some activities that you can do to lower stress are taking leisure walks, light shopping, going out of town, and having romantic dates.

Aside from lowering stress levels, you also need to remember to eat right, to get the right amount of sleep, and to avoid vices that may affect your chances of getting pregnant. You need to get the right amount of energy so that when it is time to have sexual intercourse with your partner, your body does not feel spent and all your organs are green and go.

During Sexual Intercourse

Yes, it is stated above that no particular sexual position can optimize your chances of getting pregnant however it is also true that your sexual position during ejaculation can have the direct effect on the trajectory of the semen inside the woman's cervix. Although your man ejects millions of sperms in every teaspoon of semen, you need to help his swimmers reach your fertile egg. One way to help your man's tiny army is to use gravity on your side. So go ahead and enjoy all sort of sexual position you wish to try but once it is time for ejaculation remind your man to tell you so you can raise your hips up so his semen has additional gravitational assistance towards your uterus. Even if there is no scientific basis yet for this practice, there is no harm in raising your hips about 4 inches higher than your head for 5 minutes. Just do not go to the extremes and do a head stand immediately after orgasm. It is still normal for some of the semen to drip out of the vagina but remember the more semen that enters your cervix increases the chances of conceiving.

After Sexual Intercourse

It is best to cuddle after sex. That way, your lying position will help the sperms swim faster towards your cervix. Standing up immediately after sex will drip more semen from your vagina and that is not a wise move. Cuddling also keeps your bodies aroused which mean that both your vagina and cervix are kept broader than usual. That extra space allows faster entrance of sperms to your uterus.

It is also best to rest in bed after sex so that your body can focus all its energy on what's happening internally. Getting out of bed to go back to your normal routine might just distract your body from what is more important. Finally, do not take a hot bath during and after sex because it affects the mortality of the sperms. Remember, sperms cannot take heat beyond 37°C so it will immediately weaken and kill them if you bathe in a hot tub.

Frequency of Sexual Intercourse

Another question that is frequently asked by a lot of couples is the frequency of sexual intercourse to increase chances of getting pregnant. When it comes to getting pregnant, the saying "Try and try until you succeed" may not be applicable. Your eagerness to have a "bun in the oven" should not equate to the number of times you consummate every single free time you have. You should also think of what sex does to you and your partner's bodies before you just go and do the deed anytime.

The frequency of sexual intercourse has a huge effect on men. Men who ejaculate every single day produce fewer sperms every orgasm. On the contrary, sperms die if they spend a lot of time in the testicles waiting to be ejaculated. This means that if men have sex once or twice a week only, chances are the sperms they will ejaculate already dead or about to die. Timing is key for men to produce the strongest and the most number of sperms. In line with this, men are recommended to have sex every other day to optimize the production of sperms. A day's rest enough for the male reproductive system to replenish its stock with the best quality of sperms. Once the female enter the ovulation period, these window days are the exception to the every other day rule. Have sex every day for the next few days until your ovulation period ends to increase your chances of conceiving.

Chapter 8: Congratulations! You Are Pregnant!

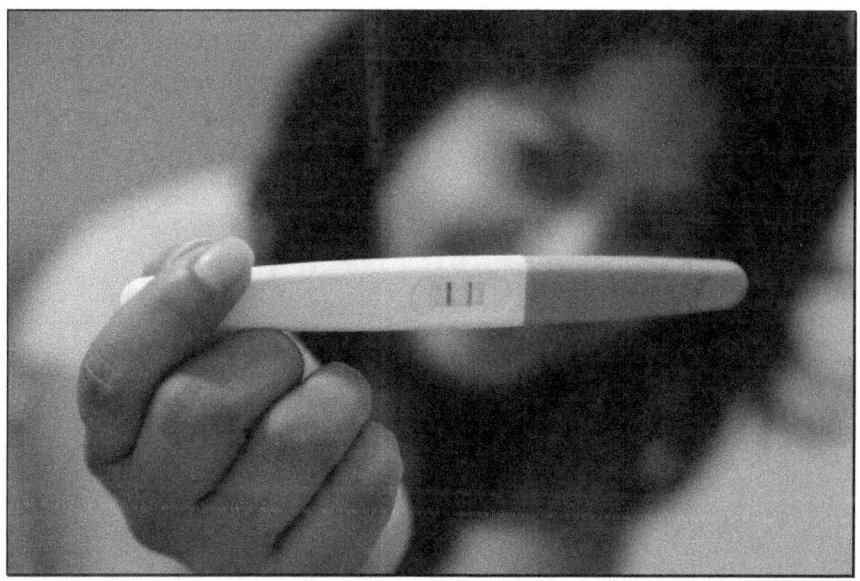

How soon can you confirm that you are pregnant? Medically speaking, one cannot confirm successful conception not until four weeks after sexual intercourse and after skipping a menstrual cycle. Here are some tell-tale signs that may indicate that you are pregnant:

- *Backache*

    As soon as the female egg is fertilized, the egg slowly moves from the fallopian tube to the uterus. Once this happens, the brain prepares the body for the inevitable changes that will happen physically and physiologically.

Due to these changes, the lower part of your back may start aching because of the expansion of the uterus. This may take effect as early as the first couple of weeks after fertilization.

- *Swollen Breasts*

You will assume that your tender breasts are due to your upcoming menstrual cycle but swollen breasts may also indicate successful fertilization. Since the brain has already sent signals that the body is growing a fetus, the mammary glands are signaled to get ready to produce enough milk in 40 weeks.

- *No Menstruation*

One of the best indication that you are pregnant is when you missed your menstruation. This is especially true for women who have regular menstrual cycles. This happens at least two weeks after sexual intercourse.

- *Morning Sickness*

Nausea or morning sickness starts six weeks after conception and lasts until the 3rd month of pregnancy. Although coined as "morning sickness," the feeling of nausea may happen morning, noon, and night. Most women go through this symptom due to the physiological changes that are occurring in the body. If you experience morning sickness, try to eat foods that do not have the intense smell and try to walk every morning to keep yourself busy.

- *Just Plain Tired*

You did not do much but you feel so tired even during the early hours of the day. The feeling of fatigue can be attributed to the body's surging hormones and the internal changes that are happening. If you feel tired, just rest for a few minutes. Do not counter the feeling because it is your body's way of telling you to take things slow.

• *Peeing All the Time*

You are taking the same amount of fluids as before but you take more frequent trips to the toilet to pee. This could be a sign that you are pregnant. The body produces more fluids during pregnancy and this can result in frequent visits to the restroom.

• *Food Cravings*

You never liked sour or salty dishes but you suddenly dream of eating sour fruits or salty snacks. This again can be a sign that you are pregnant. The sudden surge of hormones may have affected your desire to eat. It can either desensitize your palate or worse extremely sensitize your tongue.

• *Sensitive Olfactory*

You used to like your partner's cologne or perfume, but you just woke up one day with its revolting smell. Pregnancy can also affect your olfactory bulbs which are why you are very sensitive to all sorts of smell. Even some scents that cannot be noticed by other people can magically be noticed by a pregnant woman. Try to stay away from such smells so that it will not trigger your nausea.

• *Feeling Hot*

Feeling hot does not mean you feel sexy; it means you feel like being under the sun even if the temperature is normal for other people. Pregnant women normally have higher basal body temperatures, so they tend to feel hot and sweat more. To counter this annoying feeling, wear comfortable clothing.

* *Spotting*

You do not know if your menstruation has already begun because you see blood spots on your undies, but you are quite sure that it is not enough to be considered as menstruation. Pregnant women can sometimes experience spotting especially a week or two after fertilization because this is an indication that the fertilized egg has just implanted itself onto the uterus wall.

Of course, the only way you can confirm that you are really pregnant is through an abdominal ultrasound or through a pregnancy test. The latter is more convenient to do than the former; however, it is still safer to have your doctor read your ultrasound results. After all, once you get a smiley face or two lines on your pregnancy stick, you would really have to visit your doctor.

What to do during the First Trimester?

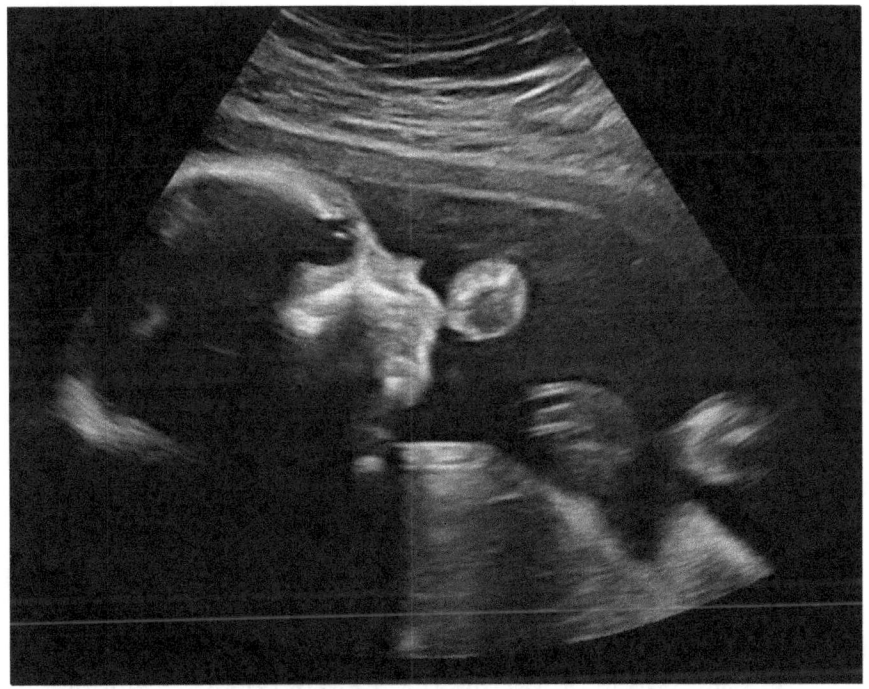

Now that your OB-GYNE has confirmed that you are indeed pregnant, what should you do to protect your growing fetus as well as yourself?

- *Religiously take your vitamins*

  Most definitely, your OB-GYNE has prescribed you some supplements or vitamins to ensure the healthy development of your soon-to-be bundle of joy. Since you are now sharing your nutrients to your baby, you need these supplements and vitamins so that your body will not feel weak and more importantly your baby will not be underdeveloped. Pregnant women still need a lot of Folic Acid so ask your doctor what dose you need to take.

- *Choose the right OB-GYNE*

If you still do not have an OB-GYNE, it is important that you choose the right one for your needs. You will make frequent visits to this doctor so you need to select one who patiently answers your questions, willing to listen to your requests, and honest enough to tell you what you should and should not do.

- *Eat healthy*

If you balanced your diet to prepare for pregnancy, then you need to be even more careful now that you are eating for two. Eat foods that are rich in folate, calcium, iron, and zinc because these are what your body needs to healthily develop your baby. Aside from these vitamin-rich foods, you also need to consume enough fiber to prevent any constipation, which is common to most pregnant women. However, do avoid food that produces gas like beans or too much lettuce because pregnant women tend to feel bloated easily.

- *Do not take "Eating for Two" literally*

Yes, you are eating for two, but this does not mean that you have to pig out every chance you get. You need to watch your weight because this can make your pregnancy either a breeze or a great obstacle. Control your intake so that you will not end up having preeclampsia or hypertension or diabetes.

- *Drink lots of water*

You need to consume at least ten glasses of water or about half a gallon every day to stay hydrated. Since your body is producing and releasing a lot more fluids, you need to replenish this by drinking water. It is better to purchase those water bottles that measure the amount of water intake so that you are constantly guided if you have taken enough water for the day.

Conclusion

The entire experience of motherhood starts a few months before getting pregnant. Every woman should take this great responsibility in stride because the gift of life is what is waiting at the end of this process. And it is only through the completion of this entire process will you feel what unconditional love is. For you to be able to give that insurmountable amount of love, you will need a lot of support and love in order to get through this phase of your life. This is where your partner comes in. From the preparation stage, pregnancy stage, childbirth stage, up to the child-rearing stage, your partner will play an important role in completing your motherhood role.